The Innovative Dash Diet Cookbook

A Collection of 50 Dishes for Weight Loss and a Fit Lifestyle

Eleonore Barlow

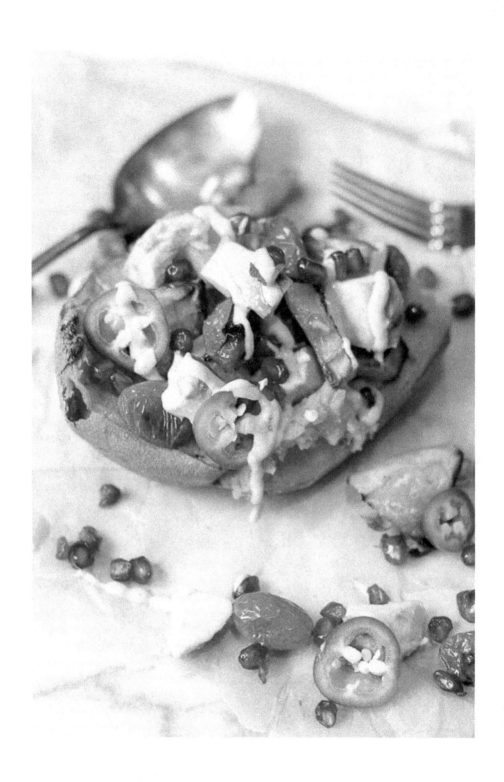

Table of Contents

Herbed Parmesan Walnuts

Serving: 4

Prep Time: 5 minutes

Cook Time: 30 minutes

Ingredients:

½ cup kite ricotta/cashew cheese

½ teaspoon Italian herb seasoning and garlic sunflower seeds

1 teaspoon parsley flakes

2 cups walnuts

1 egg white

How To:

1.   Preheat your oven to 250 degrees F.

2.   Take a bowl and add all ingredients except the albumen and walnuts.

3.   Whisk within the albumen, stir in halved walnuts and blend well.

4.   Transfer the mixture to a greased baking sheet and bake for half-hour.

5.   Serve and enjoy!

Nutrition (Per Serving)

Calories: 220

Fat: 21g

Carbohydrates: 4g

Protein 8g

Amazing Scrambled Turkey Eggs

Serving: 2

Prep Time: 15 minutes

Cook Time: 15 minutes

Ingredients:

1 tablespoon coconut oil

1 medium red bell pepper, diced

½ medium yellow onion, diced

¼ teaspoon hot pepper sauce

3 large free-range eggs

¼ teaspoon black pepper, freshly ground ¼ teaspoon salt

How To:

1.   Set a pan to medium-high heat, add copra oil, let it heat up.

2.   Add onions and sauté.

3.   Add turkey and red pepper.

4.   Cook until the turkey is cooked.

5.   Take a bowl and beat eggs, stir in salt and pepper.

6.   Pour eggs within the pan with turkey and gently cook and scramble eggs.

7.   Top with sauce and enjoy!

Nutrition (Per Serving)

Calories: 435

Fat: 30g

Carbohydrates: 34g

Protein: 16g

Egg and Bacon Cups

Serving: 6

Prep Time: 10 minutes

Cook Time: 15 minutes

Ingredients:

2 bacon strips

2 large eggs

A handful of fresh spinach

¼ cup cheese

Salt and pepper to taste

How To:

1.	Preheat your oven to 400 degrees F.

2.	Fry bacon during a skillet over medium heat, drain the oil and keep them on the side.

3.	Take muffin tin and grease with oil.

4.	Line with a slice of bacon, depress the bacon well, ensuring that the ends are protruding (to be used as handles).

5.   Take a bowl and beat eggs.

6.   Drain and pat the spinach dry.

7.   Add the spinach to the eggs.

8.   Add 1 / 4 of the mixture in each of your muffin tins.

9.   Sprinkle cheese and season.

10.   Bake for quarter-hour.

11.   Enjoy!

Nutrition (Per Serving)

Calories: 101

Fat: 7g

Carbohydrates: 2g

Protein: 8g

Fiber: 1g

Net Carbs: 1g

Pepperoni Omelet

Serving: 2

Prep Time: 5 minutes

Cook Time: 20 minutes

Ingredients:

3 eggs

7 pepperoni slices

1 teaspoon coconut cream

Salt and freshly ground black pepper, to taste 1 tablespoons butter

How To:

1.   Take a bowl and whisk eggs with all the remaining ingredients in it.

2.   Then take a skillet and warmth the butter.

3.   Pour ¼ of the egg mixture into your skillet.

4.   After that, cook for two minutes per side.

5.   Repeat to use the whole batter.

6.   Serve warm and enjoy!

Nutrition (Per Serving)

Calories: 141

Fat: 11.5g

Carbohydrates: 0.6g

Protein: 8.9g

Cinnamon Baked Apple Chips

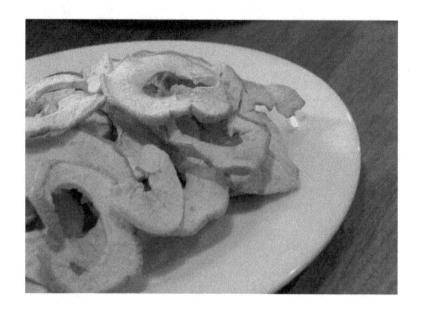

Serving: 2

Prep Time: 5 minutes

Cook Time: 2 hours

Ingredients:

1 teaspoon cinnamon

1-2 apples

How To:

1.   Preheat your oven to 200 degrees F.

2.   Take a pointy knife and slice apples into thin slices.

3.   Discard seeds.

4.   Line a baking sheet with parchment paper and arrange apples thereon.

5.   Confirm they are doing not overlap.

6.   Once done, sprinkle cinnamon over apples.

7.   Bake within the oven for 1 hour.

8.   Flip and bake for an hour more until not moist.

9.   Serve and enjoy!

Nutrition (Per Serving)

Calories: 147

Fat: 0g

Carbohydrates: 39g

Protein: 1g

Herb and Avocado Omelet

Serving: 2

Prep Time: 2 minutes

Cook Time: 10 minutes

Ingredients:

3 large free-range eggs

½ medium avocado, sliced

½ cup almonds, sliced

Salt and pepper as needed

How To:

1.	Take a non-stick skillet and place it over medium-high heat.

2.	Take a bowl and add eggs, beat the eggs.

3.	Pour into the skillet and cook for 1 minute.

4.	Reduce heat to low and cook for 4 minutes.

5.	Top the omelet with almonds and avocado.

6.   Sprinkle salt and pepper and serve.

7.   Enjoy!

Nutrition (Per Serving)

Calories: 193

Fat: 15g

Carbohydrates: 5g

Protein: 10g

Classic Apple and Cinnamon Oatmeal

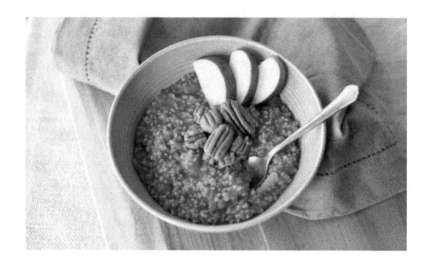

Serving: 4

Prep Time: 15 minutes

Cook Time: 7-9 hours

Ingredients:

1 apple, cored, peeled and diced

1 cup steel-cut oats

2 ½ cups unsweetened vanilla almond milk

2 tablespoons honey

½ teaspoon vanilla extract

1 teaspoon ground cinnamon

How To:

1.   Grease the Slow Cooker well.

2.   Add the listed ingredients to your Slow Cooker and stir.

3.   Cover with lid and cook on LOW for 7-9 hours.

4.   Serve and enjoy!

Nutrition (Per Serving)

Calories: 126

Fat: 3g

Carbohydrates: 25g

Protein: 3g

Blackberry Chicken Wings

Serving: 4

Prep Time: 35 minutes

Cook Time: 50minutes

Ingredients:

3 pounds chicken wings, about 20 pieces ½ cup blackberry chipotle jam Sunflower seeds and pepper to taste ½ cup water

How To:

1.   Add water and jam to a bowl and blend well.

2.   Place chicken wings during a zip bag and add two-thirds of the marinade.

3.   Season with sunflower seeds and pepper.

4.   Let it marinate for half-hour.

5.   Pre-heat your oven to 400 degrees F.

6.   Prepare a baking sheet and wire rack, place chicken wings in wire rack and bake for quarter-hour.

7.   Brush remaining marinade and bake for half-hour more.

8.   Enjoy!

Nutrition (Per Serving)

Calories: 502

Fat: 39g

Carbohydrates: 01.8g

Protein: 34g

Generous Lemon Dredged Broccoli

Serving: 4

Prep Time: 10 minutes

Cook Time: 15 minutes

Ingredients:

2 heads broccoli, separated into florets

2 teaspoons extra virgin olive oil

1 teaspoon sunflower seeds

½ teaspoon pepper

1 garlic clove, minced

½ teaspoon lemon juice

How To:

1.   Pre-heat your oven to a temperature of 400 degrees F.

2.   Take an outsized sized bowl and add broccoli florets with some extra virgin vegetable oil, pepper, sea sunflower seeds and garlic.

3.   Spread the broccoli call at one even layer on a fine baking sheet.

4.   Bake in your pre-heated oven for about 15-20 minutes until the florets are soft enough to be pierced with a fork.

5.   Squeeze juice over them generously before serving.

6.   Enjoy!

Nutrition (Per Serving)

Calories: 49

Fat: 2g

Carbohydrates: 4g

Protein: 3g

Tantalizing Almond butter Beans

Serving: 4

Prep Time: 5 minutes

Cook Time: 12 minutes

Ingredients:

2 garlic cloves, minced

Red pepper flakes to taste

Sunflower seeds to taste

2 tablespoons clarified butter

4 cups green beans, trimmed

How To:

1.   Bring a pot of water to boil, with added seeds for taste.

2.   Once the water starts to boil, add beans and cook for 3 minutes.

3.   Take a bowl of drinking water and drain beans, plunge them into the drinking water.

4.   Once cooled, keep them on the side.

5. Take a medium skillet and place it over medium heat, add ghee and melt.

6. Add red pepper, sunflower seeds, garlic.

7. Cook for 1 minute.

8. Add beans and toss until coated well, cook for 3 minutes.

9. Serve and enjoy!

Nutrition (Per Serving)

Calories: 93

Fat: 8g

Carbohydrates: 4g

Protein: 2g

Healthy Chicken Cream Salad

Serving: 3

Prep Time: 5 minutes

Cook Time: 50 minutes

Ingredients:

2 chicken breasts

1 ½ cups low fat cream

3 ounces celery

2-ounce green pepper, chopped

½ ounce green onion, chopped

½ cup low fat mayo

3 hard-boiled eggs, chopped

How To:

1.   Pre-heat your oven to 350 degrees F.

2.   Take a baking sheet and place chicken, cover with cream.

3.   Bake for 30-40 minutes.

4.   Take a bowl and blend within the chopped celery, peppers, onions.

5.   Chop the baked chicken into bite-sized portions.

6.   Peel and chop the hard-boiled eggs.

7.   · Take an outsized salad bowl and blend in eggs, veggies and chicken.

8.   Toss well and serve.

9.   Enjoy!

Nutrition (Per Serving)

Calories: 415

Fat: 24g

Carbohydrates: 4g

Protein: 40g

Generously Smothered Pork Chops

Serving: 4

Prep Time: 10 minutes

Cook Time: 30 minutes

Ingredients:

4 pork chops, bone-in

2 tablespoons of olive oil

¼ cup vegetable broth

½ pound Yukon gold potatoes, peeled and chopped 1 large onion, sliced

2 garlic cloves, minced

2 teaspoon rubbed sage

1 teaspoon thyme, ground

Pepper as needed

How To:

1.   Pre-heat your oven to 350 degrees F.

2.   Take an outsized sized skillet and place it over medium heat.

3.   Add a tablespoon of oil and permit the oil to heat up.

4.   Add pork chops and cook them for 4-5 minutes per side until browned.

5.   Transfer chops to a baking dish.

6.   Pour broth over the chops.

7.   Add remaining oil to the pan and sauté potatoes, onion, garlic for 3-4 minutes.

8.   Take an outsized bowl and add potatoes, garlic, onion, thyme, sage, pepper.

9.   Transfer this mixture to the baking dish (wish pork).

10.   Bake for 20-30 minutes.

11.   Serve and enjoy!

Nutrition (Per Serving)

Calorie: 261

Fat: 10g

Carbohydrates: 1.3g

Protein: 2g

Black Eyed Peas and Spinach Platter

Serving: 4

Prep Time: 10 minutes

Cook Time: 8 hours

Ingredients:

1 cup black eyed peas, soaked overnight and drained

2 cups low-sodium vegetable broth

1 can (15 ounces) tomatoes, diced with juice

8 ounces ham, chopped

1 onion, chopped

2 garlic cloves, minced

1 teaspoon dried oregano

1 teaspoon salt

½ teaspoon freshly ground black pepper ½ teaspoon ground mustard 1 bay leaf

How To:

1.   Add the listed ingredients to your Slow Cooker and stir.

2.   Place lid and cook on LOW for 8 hours.

3.   Discard the herb.

4.   Serve and enjoy!

Nutrition (Per Serving)

Calories: 209

Fat: 6g

Carbohydrates: 22g

Protein: 17g

Humble Mushroom Rice

Serving: 3

Prep Time: 10 minutes

Cook Time: 3 hours

Ingredients:

½ cup rice

2 green onions chopped

1 garlic clove, minced

¼ pound baby Portobello mushrooms, sliced 1 cup vegetable stock

How To:

1.   Add rice, onions, garlic, mushrooms, stock to your Slow Cooker.

2.   Stir well and place lid.

3.   Cook on LOW for 3 hours.

4.   Stir and divide amongst serving platters.

5. Enjoy!

Nutrition (Per Serving)

Calories: 200

Fat: 6g

Carbohydrates: 28g

Protein: 5g

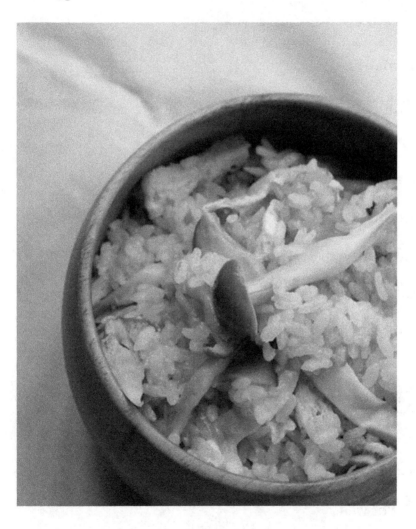

Sweet and Sour Cabbage and Apples

Serving: 4

Prep Time: 15 minutes

Cook Time: 8 hours

Ingredients:

¼ cup honey

¼ cup apple cider vinegar

2 tablespoons Orange Chili-Garlic Sauce

1 teaspoon sea salt

3 sweet tart apples, peeled, cored and sliced

2 heads green cabbage, cored and shredded

1 sweet red onion, thinly sliced

How To:

1.   Take a little bowl and whisk in honey, orange-chili aioli , vinegar.

2.   Stir well.

3. Add honey mix, apples, onion and cabbage to your Slow Cooker and stir.

4. Close lid and cook on LOW for 8 hours.

5. Serve and enjoy!

Nutrition (Per Serving)

Calories: 164

Fat: 1g

Carbohydrates: 41g

Protein: 4g

Delicious Aloo Palak

Serving: 6

Prep Time: 10 minutes

Cook Time: 6-8 hours

Ingredients:

2 pounds red potatoes, chopped

1 small onion, diced

1 red bell pepper, seeded and diced

¼ cup fresh cilantro, chopped

1/3 cup low-sodium veggie broth

1 teaspoon salt

½ teaspoon Garam masala

½ teaspoon ground cumin

¼ teaspoon ground turmeric

¼ teaspoon ground coriander

¼ teaspoon freshly ground black pepper 2 pounds fresh spinach, chopped

How To:

1.   Add potatoes, bell pepper, onion, cilantro, broth and seasoning to your Slow Cooker.

2.   Mix well.

3.   Add spinach on top.

4.   Place lid and cook on LOW for 6-8 hours.

5.   Stir and serve.

6.   Enjoy!

Nutrition (Per Serving)

Calories: 205

Fat: 1g

Carbohydrates: 44g

Protein: 9g

Healthy Mediterranean Lamb Chops

Serving: 4

Prep Time: 10 minutes

Cook Time: 10-minute

Ingredients:

4 lamb shoulder chops, 8 ounces each

2 tablespoons Dijon mustard

2 tablespoons Balsamic vinegar

½ cup olive oil

2 tablespoons shredded fresh basil

How To:

1.   Pat your lamb chops dry using a kitchen towel and arrange them on a shallow glass baking dish.

2.   Take a bowl and whisk in Dijon mustard, balsamic vinegar, pepper and mix them well.

3.   Whisk in the oil very slowly into the marinade until the mixture is smooth.

4. Stir in basil.

5. Pour the marinade over the lamb chops and stir to coat both sides well.

6. Cover the chops and allow them to marinate for 1-4 hours (chilled).

7. Take the chops out and let them rest for 30 minutes to allow the temperature to reach a normal level.

8. Pre-heat your grill to medium heat and add oil to the grate.

9. Grill the lamb chops for 5-10 minutes per side until both sides are browned.

10. Once the center reads 145 degrees F, the chops are ready, serve and enjoy!

Nutrition (Per Serving)

Calories: 521

Fat: 45g

Carbohydrates: 3.5g

Protein: 22g

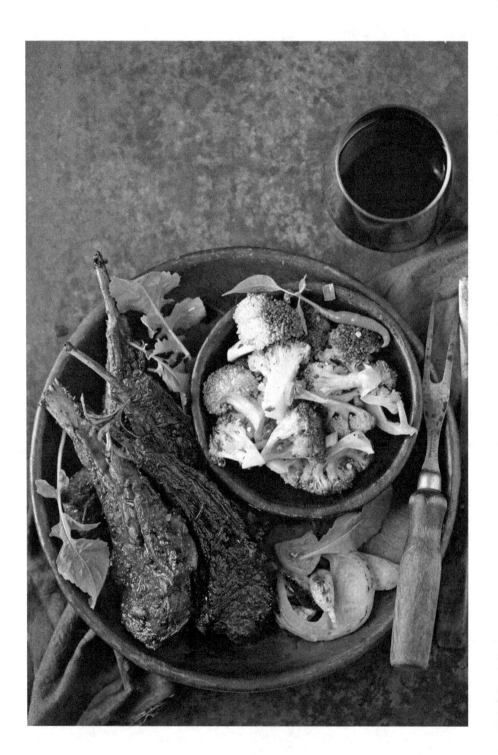

A Turtle Friend Salad

Serving: 6

Prep Time: 5 minutes

Cook Time: 5 minutes

Ingredients:

1 Romaine lettuce, chopped

3 Roma tomatoes, diced

1 English cucumber, diced

1 small red onion, diced

½ cup parsley, chopped

2 tablespoons virgin olive oil

½ large lemon, juice

1 teaspoon garlic powder

Sunflower seeds and pepper to taste

How To:

1. Wash the vegetables thoroughly under cold water.

2. Prepare them by chopping, dicing or mincing as needed.

3. Take a large salad bowl and transfer the prepped veggies.

4. Add vegetable oil, olive oil, lemon juice, and spice.

5. Toss well to coat.

6. Serve chilled if preferred.

7. Enjoy!

Nutrition (Per Serving)

Calories: 200

Fat: 8g

Carbohydrates: 18g

Protein: 10g

Avocado and Cilantro Mix

Serving: 2

Prep Time: 10 minutes

Cook Time: nil

Ingredients:

2 avocados, peeled, pitted and diced

1 sweet onion, chopped

1 green bell pepper, chopped

1 large ripe tomato, chopped

¼ cup of fresh cilantro, chopped

½ lime, juiced

Sunflower seeds and pepper as needed

How To:

1.   Take a medium sized bowl and add onion, tomato, avocados, bell pepper, lime and cilantro.

2.   Give the whole mixture a toss.

3.   Season accordingly and serve chilled.

4.   Enjoy!

Nutrition (Per Serving)

Calories: 126

Fat: 10g

Carbohydrates: 10g

Protein: 2g

Exceptional Watercress and Melon Salad

Serving: 4

Prep Time: 15 minutes

Cook Time: 20 minutes

Ingredients:

3 tablespoons lime juice

1 teaspoon date paste

1 teaspoon fresh ginger root, minced

¼ cup vegetable oil

2 bunch watercress, chopped

2 ½ cups watermelon, cubed

2 ½ cups cantaloupe, cubed

1/3 cup almonds, toasted and sliced

How To:

1.   Take a large sized bowl and add lime juice, ginger, date paste.

2.   Whisk well and add oil.

3.   Season with pepper and sunflower seeds.

4.   Add watercress, watermelon.

5.   Toss well

6.   Transfer to a serving bowl and garnish with sliced almonds.

7.   Enjoy!

Nutrition (Per Serving)

Calories: 274

Fat: 20g

Carbohydrates: 21g

Protein: 7g

Zucchini and Onions Platter

Serving: 4

Prep Time: 15 minutes

Cook Time: 45 minutes

Ingredients:

3 large zucchini, julienned

1 cup cherry tomatoes, halved

½ cup basil

2 red onions, thinly sliced

¼ teaspoon sunflower seeds

1 teaspoon cayenne pepper

2 tablespoons lemon juice

How To:

1.   Create zucchini Zoodles by using a vegetable peeler and shaving the zucchini with peeler lengthwise until you get to the core and seeds.

2.   Turn zucchini and repeat until you have long strips.

3. Discard seeds.

4. Lay strips in cutting board and slice lengthwise to your desired thickness.

5. Mix Zoodles in a bowl alongside onion, basil, tomatoes and toss.

6. Sprinkle sunflower seeds and cayenne pepper on top.

7. Drizzle lemon juice.

8. Serve and enjoy!

Nutrition (Per Serving)

Calories: 156

Fat: 8g

Carbohydrates: 6g

Protein: 7g

Tender Watermelon and Radish Salad

Serving: 4

Prep Time: 15 minutes

Cook Time: 25 minutes

Ingredients:

medium beets, peeled and cut into 1-inch chunks 1 teaspoon extra virgin olive oil 4 cups seedless watermelon, diced

1 tablespoon fresh thyme, chopped

1 lemon, juiced

2 cups kale, torn

3 cups radish, diced

Sunflower seeds, to taste

Pepper, to taste

How To:

1.   Pre-heat your oven to 350 degrees F.

2.   Take a small bowl and add beets, olive oil and toss well to coat the beets.

3.   Roast beets for 25 minutes until tender.

4.   Transfer to large bowl and cool them.

5.   Add watermelon, kale, radishes, thyme, lemon juice, and toss.

6.   Season sea sunflower seeds and pepper.

7.   Serve and enjoy!

Nutrition (Per Serving)

Calories: 178

Fat: 2g

Carbohydrates: 39g

Protein: 6g

Fiery Tomato Salad

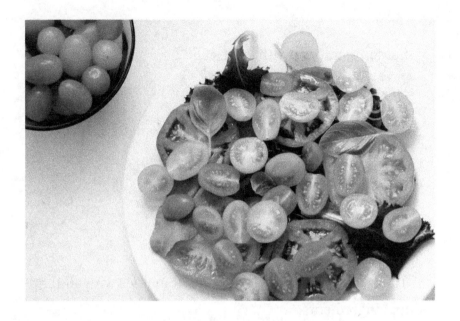

Serving: 4

Prep Time: 10 minutes

Cook Time: 25 minutes

Ingredients:

½ cup scallions, chopped

1 pound cherry tomatoes

3 teaspoons olive oil

Sea sunflower seeds and freshly ground black pepper, to taste 1 tablespoon red wine vinegar

How To:

1.   Season tomatoes with spices and oil.

2.   Heat your oven to 450 degrees F.

3.   Take a baking sheet and spread the tomatoes.

4.   Bake for 15 minutes.

5.   Stir and turn the tomatoes.

6.   Then, bake again for 10 minutes.

7.   Take a bowl and mix the roasted tomatoes with all the remaining ingredients.

8.   Serve and enjoy!

Nutrition (Per Serving)

Calories: 115

Fat: 10.4g

Carbohydrates: 5.4g

Protein: 12g

Spiced Up Salmon

Serving: 4

Prep Time: 10 minutes

Cook Time: 10 minutes

Ingredients:

Salmon fillets

2 tablespoons olive oil

1 teaspoon cumin, ground

1 teaspoon sweet paprika

1 teaspoon chili powder

½ teaspoon garlic powder

Pinch of pepper

How To:

1.   Take a bowl and add cumin, paprika, onion, chili powder, garlic powder, pepper and toss well.

2.   Rub the salmon in the mixture.

3.   Take a pan and place it over medium heat, add oil and let it heat up.

4.   Add salmon and cook for 5 minutes, both sides.

5.   Divide between plates and serve.

6.   Enjoy!

Nutrition (Per Serving)

Calories: 220

Fat: 10g

Net Carbohydrates: 8g

Protein: 10g

Coconut Cream Shrimp

Serving: 4

Prep Time: 10 minutes

Cook Time: nil

Ingredients:

1 pound shrimp, cooked, peeled and deveined

1 tablespoon coconut cream

¼ teaspoon jalapeno, chopped ½ teaspoon lime juice 1 tablespoon parsley, chopped Pinch of pepper

How To:

1.   Take a bowl and add shrimp, cream, jalapeno, lime juice, parsley, pepper.

2.   Toss well and divide into small bowls.

3.   Serve and enjoy!

Nutrition (Per Serving)

Calories: 183

Fat: 5g

Net Carbohydrates: 12g

Protein: 8g

Shrimp and Avocado Platter

Serving: 8

Prep Time: 10 minutes

Cook Time: nil

Ingredients:

2 green onions, chopped

2 avocados, pitted, peeled and cut into chunks

2 tablespoons cilantro, chopped

1 cup shrimp, cooked, peeled and deveined Pinch of pepper

How To:

1.　　Take a bowl and add cooked shrimp, avocado, green onions, cilantro, pepper.

2.　　Toss well and serve.

3.　　Enjoy!

Nutrition (Per Serving)

Calories: 160

Fat: 2g

Net Carbohydrates: 5g

Protein: 6g

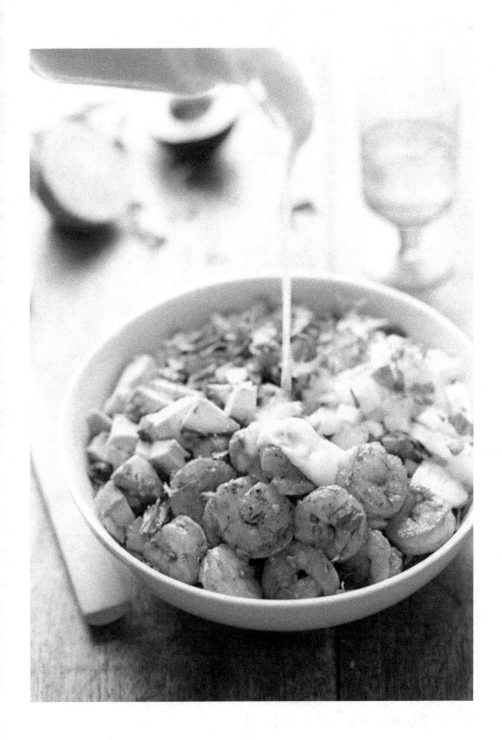

Calamari

Serving: 4

Prep Time: 10 minutes +1-hour marinating

Cook Time: 8 minutes

Ingredients:

2 tablespoons extra virgin olive oil

1 teaspoon chili powder

½ teaspoon ground cumin

Zest of 1 lime

Juice of 1 lime

Dash of sea sunflower seeds

½ pounds squid, cleaned and split open, with tentacles cut into ½ inch rounds

tablespoons cilantro, chopped

tablespoons red bell pepper, minced

How To:

1.   Take a medium bowl and stir in olive oil, chili powder, cumin, lime zest, sea sunflower seeds, lime juice and pepper.

2.   Add squid and let it marinade and stir to coat, coat and let it refrigerate for 1 hour

3.   Pre-heat your oven to broil.

4.   Arrange squid on a baking sheet, broil for 8 minutes turn once until tender.

5.   Garnish the broiled calamari with cilantro and red bell pepper.

6.   Serve and enjoy!

Nutrition (Per Serving)

Calories: 159

Fat: 13g

Carbohydrates: 12g

Protein: 3g

Hearty Deep-Fried Prawn and Rice Croquettes

Serving: 8

Prep Time: 25 minutes

Cook Time: 13 minutes

Ingredients:

2 tablespoons almond butter

½ onion, chopped

ounces shrimp, peeled and chopped

2 tablespoons all-purpose flour

tablespoon white wine

½ cup almond milk

tablespoons almond milk

cups cooked rice

1 tablespoon parmesan, grated

1 teaspoon fresh dill, chopped

1 teaspoon sunflower seeds

Ground pepper as needed

Vegetable oil for frying

tablespoons all-purpose flour

1 whole egg

½ cup breadcrumbs

How To:

1.   Take a large skillet and place it over medium heat, add almond butter and let it melt.

2.   Add onion, cook and stir for 5 minutes.

3.   Add shrimp and cook for 1-2 minutes.

4.   Stir in 2 tablespoons flour, white wine, pour in almond milk gradually and cook for 3-5 minutes until the sauce thickens.

5.   Remove white sauce from heat and stir in rice, mix evenly.

6.   Add parmesan, cheese, dill, sunflower seeds, pepper and let it cool for 15 minutes.

7.   Heat oil in large saucepan and bring it to 350 degrees F.

8.   Take a bowl and whisk in egg, spread breadcrumbs on a plate.

9.   Form rice mixture into 8 balls and roll 1 ball in flour, dip in egg and coat with crumbs, repeat with all balls.

10.   Deep fry balls for 3 minutes.

11.   Enjoy!

Nutrition (Per Serving)

Calories: 182

Fat: 7g

Carbohydrates: 21g

Protein: 7g

Ground Turkey Mini Meatloaves

Prep time: 10 minutes

Cook time: 30 minutes

Servings: 6

Ingredients

Lean ground turkey – 1 ½ pound

Onion – 1, diced

Celery – 2, diced

Bell pepper – 1, diced

Garlic – 4 cloves, minced

No-salt-added tomato sauce – 1 (8-ounce) can Egg white – 1

Salt-free bread crumbs – ¾ cup Molasses – 1 Tbsp.

Liquid smoke – ¼ tsp.

Freshly ground black pepper - ½ tsp. Salt-free ketchup – ¼ cup

Method

1.   Preheat the oven to 375F. Spray a 6-cup muffin tin with oil and set aside.

2.   Place all ingredients except for ketchup in a bowl and mix well.

3.   Fill the muffin cups with the mixture and press in firmly.

4.   Divide the ketchup between the muffin cups and spread evenly.

5.   Place muffin tin on the middle rack in the oven and bake for 30 minutes.

6.   Remove, cool, and serve.

Nutritional Facts Per Serving

Calories: 251

Fat: 7g

Carb: 21g

Protein: 25g

Sodium 112mg

Turkey and Brown Rice Stuffed Peppers

Prep time: 10 minutes

Cook time: 35 minutes

Servings: 4

Ingredients

Bell peppers – 4, core and seeded, leave the peppers intact

Lean ground turkey – 1 pound

Onion – 1, diced

Garlic – 3 cloves, minced

Celery – 2 stalks, diced

Cooked brown rice – 2 cups

No-salt-added diced tomatoes – 1 (15-ounce) can Salt-free tomato

paste – 2 Tbsp.

Seedless raisins – ¼ cup Ground cumin – 2 tsp.

Dried oregano – 1 tsp.

Ground cinnamon – ½ tsp.

Ground black pepper – ½ tsp.

Method

1.   Preheat the oven to 425F. Grease a baking pan with oil.

2.   Heat a pan over medium heat.

3.   Add onion, ground turkey, garlic, and celery and sauté for 5 minutes. Remove from heat.

4.   Add the remaining ingredients and mix.

5.   Fill each pepper with ¼ of the mixture. Pressing firmly to pack.

6.   Stand peppers in the prebaked baking pan, replace the pepper caps and then cover the pan with foil.

7.   Place in the middle rack in the oven and bake for 25 to 30 minutes, or until tender.

8.   Serve.

Nutritional Facts Per Serving

Calories: 354

Fat: 8g

Carb: 45g

Protein: 27g

Sodium 126mg

Grilled Tequila Chicken with Peppers

Prep time: 10 minutes

Cook time: 30 minutes

Servings: 4

Ingredientes

Lime juice – 1 cup

Tequila – 1/3 cup

Garlic – 3 cloves, chopped

Chopped fresh cilantro – ¼ cup

Agave nectar – 1 Tbsp.

Ground black pepper - ½ tsp.

Cumin – 1 tsp.

Ground coriander – ½ tsp.

Boneless, skinless chicken breasts – 4

Olive oil – 2 tsp.

Green bell pepper – 1, diced

Red bell pepper – 1, diced

Onion – 1, diced

Non-fat sour cream – ½ cup

Method

1.   In a bowl, add the lime juice, tequila garlic, cilantro, agave nectar, black pepper, cumin, and coriander and mix well.

2.   Add the chicken breasts and coat well. Cover and marinate in the for least 6 hours (in the refrigerator).

3.   Heat the grill. Cook the chicken for 10 to 15 minutes per side, or no longer pink.

4.   Meanwhile, heat the oil in a pan.

5.   Add the pepper and onion. Stir-fry for 5 minutes. Remove from heat. Remove chicken from grill.

6.   Serve with veggies and sour cream.

Nutritional Facts Per Serving

Calories: 259

Fat: 3g

Carb: 18g

Protein: 28g

Sodium 118mg

Orange-Rosemary Roasted Chicken

Prep time: 10 minutes

Cook time: 45 minutes

Servings: 6

Ingredients

Chicken breast halves – 3, skinless, bone-in, each 8 ounces
Chicken legs with thigh pieces – 3, skinless, bone-in, each 8 ounces

Garlic cloves – 2, minced Extra-virgin olive oil – 1 ½ tsp.

Fresh rosemary – 3 tsp.

Ground black pepper – 1/8 tsp.

Orange juice – ½ cup

Method

1.   Preheat oven at 450F. Grease a baking pan with cooking spray.

2.   Rub chicken with garlic, then with oil. Sprinkle with pepper and rosemary.

3.   Place the chicken pieces in the baking dish.

4.   Pour the orange juice.

5.   Cover and bake for 30 minutes, then flip the chicken with tongs and cook 10 to 15 minutes more or until browned. Baste the chicken with the pan juice from time to time.

6.   Serve chicken with pan juice.

Nutritional Facts Per Serving

Calories: 204

Fat: 8g

Carb: 2g

Protein: 31g

Sodium 95mg

Honey Crusted Chicken

Prep time: 10 minutes

Cook time: 25 minutes

Servings: 2

Ingredients

Saltine crackers – 8, (2-inch square each) crushed Paprika – 1 tsp.

Chicken breasts – 2, boneless, skinless (4-ounce each)

Honey – 4 tsp.

Cooking spray to grease a baking sheet

Method

1.   Preheat the oven to 375F.

2.   In a bowl, mix crushed crackers and paprika. Mix well.

3.   In another bowl, add honey and chicken. Coat well.

4.   Add to the cracker mixture and coat well.

5.   Place the chicken in the prepared baking sheet.

6.   Bake for 20 to 25 minutes.

7.   Serve.

Nutritional Facts Per Serving

Calories: 219

Fat: 3g

Carb: 21g

Protein: 27g

Sodium 187mg

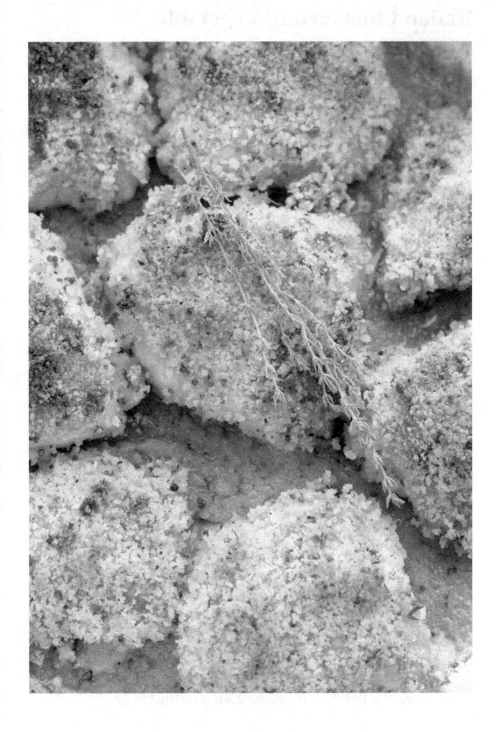

Italian Chicken and Vegetable

Prep time: 10 minutes

Cook time: 45 minutes

Servings: 1

Ingredients

Chicken breast – 1 skinless, boneless (3 ounces)

Diced zucchini – ½ cup

Diced potato – ½ cup

Diced onion – ¼ cup

Sliced baby carrots – ¼ cup

Sliced mushrooms – ¼ cup

Garlic powder – 1/8 tsp.

Italian seasoning – ¼ tsp.

Method

1.   Preheat oven to 350F.

2.   Grease a parchment paper with cooking spray.

3.   On the foil, add chicken, top mushrooms, carrots, onion, potato, and zucchini. Sprinkle with Italian seasoning and garlic powder.

4.   Fold the foil to make a packet.

5.   Place the packet on a cookie sheet.

6.   Bake until chicken and vegetables are tender, about 45 minutes.

7.   Serve.

Nutritional Facts Per Serving

Calories: 207

Fat: 2.5g

Carb: 23g

Protein: 23g

Sodium 72mg

Corn Spread

Serving: 4

Prep Time: 10 minutes

Cook Time: 10 minutes

Ingredients:

30-ounce canned corn, drained

2 green onions, chopped

½ cup coconut cream

1 jalapeno, chopped

½ teaspoon chili powder

How To:

1.   Take a pan and add corn, green onions, jalapeno, chili powder, stir well.

2.   Bring to a simmer over medium heat and cook for 10 minutes.

3.   Let it chill and add coconut cream.

4.   Stir well.

5.   Serve and enjoy!

Nutrition (Per Serving)

Calories: 192

Fat: 5g

Carbohydrates: 11g

Protein: 8g

Moroccan Leeks Snack

Serving: 4

Prep Time: 10 minutes

Cook Time: nil

Ingredients:

1 bunch radish, sliced

3 cups leeks, chopped

1 ½ cups olives, pitted and sliced

Pinch turmeric powder

2 tablespoons essential olive oil

1 cup cilantro, chopped

How To:

1.   Take a bowl and mix in radishes, leeks, olives and cilantro.

2.   Mix well.

3.   Season with pepper, oil, turmeric and toss well.

4.   Serve and enjoy!

Nutrition (Per Serving)

Calories: 120

Fat: 1g

Carbohydrates: 1g

Protein: 6g

The Bell Pepper Fiesta

Serving: 4

Prep Time: 10 minutes

Cook Time: nil

Ingredients:

2 tablespoons dill, chopped

1 yellow onion, chopped

1 pound multi colored peppers, cut, halved, seeded and cut into thin strips

3 tablespoons organic olive oil

2 ½ tablespoons white wine vinegar Black pepper to taste

How To:

1.   Take a bowl and mix in sweet pepper, onion, dill, pepper, oil, vinegar and toss well.

2.   Divide between bowls and serve.

3.   Enjoy!

Nutrition (Per Serving)

Calories: 120

Fat: 3g

Carbohydrates: 1g

Protein: 6g

Spiced Up Pumpkin Seeds Bowls

Serving: 4

Prep Time: 10 minutes

Cook Time: 20 minutes

Ingredients:

½ tablespoon chili powder

½ teaspoon cayenne

2 cups pumpkin seeds

2 teaspoons lime juice

How To:

1.   Spread pumpkin seeds over lined baking sheet, add lime juice, cayenne and chili powder.

2.   Toss well.

3.   Pre-heat your oven to 275 degrees F.

4.   Roast in your oven for 20 minutes and transfer to small bowls.

5.   Serve and enjoy!

Nutrition (Per Serving)

Calories: 170

Fat: 3g

Carbohydrates: 10g

Protein: 6g

Mozzarella Cauliflower Bars

Serving: 4

Prep Time: 10 minutes

Cook Time: 40 minutes

Ingredients:

1 cauliflower head, riced

12 cup low-fat mozzarella cheese, shredded ¼ cup egg whites

1 teaspoon Italian dressing, low fat Pepper to taste

How To:

1. Spread cauliflower rice over lined baking sheet.

2. Pre-heat your oven to 375 degrees F.

3. Roast for 20 minutes.

4. Transfer to bowl and spread pepper, cheese, seasoning, egg whites and stir well.

5. Spread in a rectangular pan and press.

6. Transfer to oven and cook for 20 minutes more.

7. Serve and enjoy!

Nutrition (Per Serving)

Calories: 140

Fat: 2g

Carbohydrates: 6g

Protein: 6g

Tomato Pesto Crackers

Serving: 4

Prep Time: 10 minutes

Cook Time: 15 minutes

Ingredients:

1 ¼ cups almond flour

½ teaspoon garlic powder

½ teaspoon baking powder

2 tablespoons sun-dried tomato Pesto

3 tablespoons ghee

½ teaspoon dried basil

¼ teaspoon pepper

How To:

1.   Pre-heat your oven to 325 degrees F.

2.   Take a bowl and add listed ingredients.

3.   Mix well and combine.

4.   Take a baking sheet lined with parchment paper and spread the dough.

5.   Transfer to oven and bake for 15 minutes. 6. Break into small sized crackers and serve.

6.   Enjoy!

Nutrition (Per Serving)

Calories: 204

Fat: 20g

Carbohydrates: 3g

Protein: 3g

Green Delight

Serving: 1

Prep Time: 10 minutes

Ingredients:

¾ cup whole almond milk yogurt

2 ½ cups lettuce mix salad greens

1 pack stevia

1 tablespoon MCT oil

1 tablespoon chia seeds

1 ½ cups water

How To:

1. Add listed ingredients to blender.
2. Blend until you have a smooth and creamy texture.
3. Serve chilled and enjoy!

Nutrition (Per Serving)

Calories: 320

Fat: 24g

Carbohydrates: 17g

Protein: 10g

Guilt Free Lemon and Rosemary Drink

Serving: 1

Prep Time: 10 minutes

Ingredients:

½ cup whole almond milk yogurt

1 cup garden greens

1 pack stevia

1 tablespoon olive oil

1 stalk fresh rosemary

1 tablespoon lemon juice, fresh

1 tablespoon pepitas

1 tablespoon flaxseed, ground

1 ½ cups water

How To:

1.　　Add listed ingredients to blender.

2.　　Blend until you have a smooth and creamy texture.

3.　　Serve chilled and enjoy!

Nutrition (Per Serving)

Calories: 312

Fat: 25g

Carbohydrates: 14g

Protein: 9g

Strawberry and Rhubarb Smoothie

Serving: 1

Prep Time: 5 minutes

Cook Time: 3 minutes

Ingredients:

1 rhubarb stalk, chopped

1 cup fresh strawberries, sliced

½ cup plain Greek strawberries

Pinch of ground cinnamon

3 ice cubes

How To:

1.   Take a small saucepan and fill with water over high heat.

2.   Bring to boil and add rhubarb, boil for 3 minutes.

3.   Drain and transfer to a blender.

4.   Add strawberries, honey, yogurt, cinnamon and pulse mixture until smooth.

5.   Add ice cubes and blend until thick with no lumps.

6.   Pour into glass and enjoy chilled.

Nutrition (Per Serving)

Calories: 295

Fat: 8g

Carbohydrates: 56g

Protein: 6g

Vanilla Hemp Drink

Serving: 1

Prep Time: 10 minutes

Ingredients:

1 cup water

1 cup unsweetened hemp almond milk, vanilla

1 ½ tablespoons coconut oil, unrefined

½ cup frozen blueberries, mixed

4 cups leafy greens, kale and spinach

1 tablespoon flaxseeds

1 tablespoon almond butter

How To:

1.   Add listed ingredients to blender.

2.   Blend until you have a smooth and creamy texture.

3.   Serve chilled and enjoy!

Nutrition (Per Serving)

Calories: 250

Fat: 20g

Carbohydrates: 10g

Protein: 7g

Yogurt and Kale Smoothie

Serving: 1

Prep Time: 10 minutes

Ingredients:

1 cup whole almond milk yogurt

1 cup baby kale greens

1 pack stevia

1 tablespoon MCT oil

1 tablespoons sunflower seeds

1 cup water

How To:

1.   Add listed ingredients to blender 2. Blend until you have a smooth and creamy texture

2.   Serve chilled and enjoy!

Nutrition (Per Serving)

Calories: 329

Fat: 26g

Carbohydrates: 15g

Protein: 11g

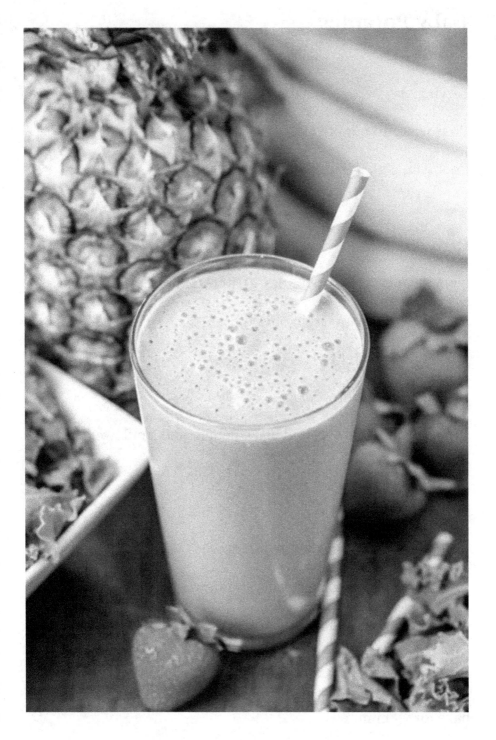

Baby Potatoes

Serving: 4

Prep Time: 10 minutes

Cook Time: 35 minutes

Ingredients:

2 pounds new yellow potatoes, scrubbed and cut into wedges

2 tablespoons extra virgin olive oil

2 teaspoons fresh rosemary, chopped

1 teaspoon garlic powder

½ teaspoon freshly ground black pepper and sunflower seeds

How To:

1.   Pre-heat your oven to 400 degrees F.

2.   Line a baking sheet with aluminum foil and set it aside.

3.   Take a large bowl and add potatoes, olive oil, garlic, rosemary, sea sunflower seeds and pepper.

4.   Spread potatoes in a single layer on a baking sheet and bake for 35 minutes.

5.   Serve and enjoy!

Nutrition (Per Serving)

Calories: 225

Fat: 7g

Carbohydrates: 37g

Protein: 5g

Cauliflower Cakes

Serving: 4

Prep Time: 10 minutes

Cook Time: 10 minutes

Ingredients:

4 cups cauliflowers, cut into florets

1 cup kite ricotta/cashew cheese, grated

2 eggs, lightly beaten

1 teaspoon paprika

1 teaspoon chili powder

Sunflower seeds and pepper to taste

½ cup fresh parsley, chopped

1 tablespoon olive oil

How To:

1.   Add cauliflower, cheese, paprika, eggs, chili, sunflower seeds, pepper and parsley into a large sized bowl.

2.   Mix well.

3.   Drizzle olive oil into frying pan and place over medium-high heat.

4.   Shape cauliflower mixture into 12 even patties.

5.   Once oil is hot, fry cakes until both sides are golden brown.

6.   Serve hot and enjoy!

Nutrition (Per Serving)

Calories: 180

Fat: 8g

Carbohydrates: 6g

Protein: 8g

Tender Coconut and Cauliflower Rice with Chili

Serving: 4

Prep Time: 20 minutes

Cook Time: 20 minutes

Ingredients:

3 cups cauliflower, riced

2/3 cups full-fat coconut almond milk

1-2 teaspoons sriracha paste

¼- ½ teaspoon onion powder

Sunflower seeds as needed

Fresh basil for garnish

How To:

1.   Take a pan and place it over medium low heat.

2.   Add all of the ingredients and stir them until fully combined.

3. Cook for about 5-10 minutes, making sure that the lid is on.

4. Remove the lid and keep cooking until any excess liquid is absorbed.

5. Once the rice is soft and creamy, enjoy!

Nutrition (Per Serving)

Calories: 95

Fat: 7g

Carbohydrates: 4g

Protein: 1g

Apple Slices

Serving: 4

Prep Time: 10 minutes

Cook Time: 10 minutes

Ingredients:

1 cup of coconut oil

¼ cup date paste

2 tablespoons ground cinnamon

4 Granny Smith apples, peeled and sliced, cored

How To:

1. Take a large sized skillet and place it over medium heat.

2. Add oil and allow the oil to heat up.

3. Stir cinnamon and date paste into the oil.

4. Add sliced apples and cook for 5-8 minutes until crispy.

5. Serve and enjoy!

Nutrition (Per Serving)

Calories: 368

Fat: 23g

Carbohydrates: 44g

Protein: 1g

The Exquisite Spaghetti Squash

Serving: 6

Prep Time: 5 minutes

Cooking Time: 7-8 hours

Ingredients:

1 spaghetti squash

2 cups water

How To:

1.   Wash squash carefully with water and rinse it well.

2.   Puncture 5-6 holes in the squash using a fork.

3.   Place squash in Slow Cooker.

4.   Place lid and cook on LOW for 7-8 hours.

5.   Remove squash to cutting board and let it cool.

6.   Cut squash in half and discard seeds.

7.   Use two forks and scrape out squash strands and transfer to bowl.

8.   Serve and enjoy!

Nutrition (Per Serving)

Calories: 52

Fat: 0g

Carbohydrates: 12g

Protein: 1g

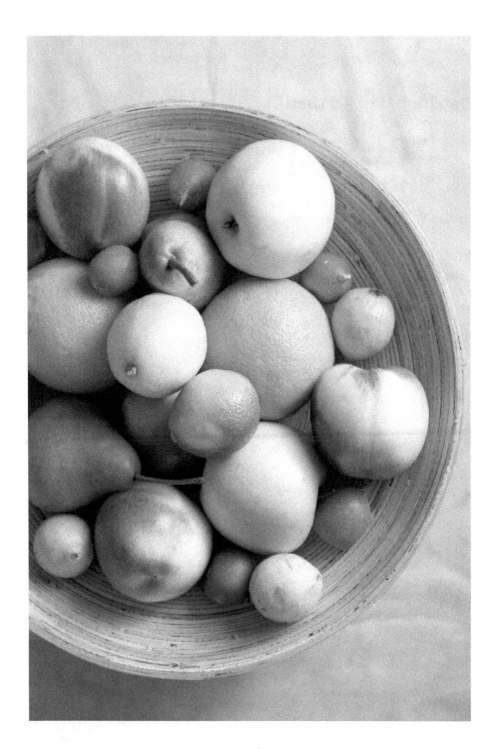

CPSIA information can be obtained
at www.ICGtesting.com
Printed in the USA
BVHW081129140521
607268BV00001B/293

9 781801 905053